# Choosing Single Parenthood: Stories from Solo Parents by Choice

COMPILED BY MALI BAIN

Choosing Single Parenthood: Stories from Solo Parents by Choice
Mali Bain, ed.
ISBN 978-1-990543-01-2
Copyright © 2021 NextGen Story: Custom Publishing

All rights reserved for collective work. Copyright of individual essays is retained by contributors.

Front cover image by Olya Sweets.

Front cover and interior design by Cara Bain.

Published by NextGen Story: Custom Publishing.
www.nextgenstory.com

# Acknowledgements

*This anthology has been a collaborative effort from the get-go.*

*Thanks to my sister Sarah, who encouraged me to move ahead with this very personal undertaking.*

*Thank you to the many people in related Facebook groups who contributed ideas, connections, and support throughout the course of this project.*

*Thanks to the volunteer editors – Barbra, Marija, Nadia, Amalie, and Zoë Sehn. Thank you to Elena Lemeneva for copy-editing each story, to David Holmes for copy-editing the entire work, and to Nadia and Marija for their final review.*

*My biggest thanks of all to those who have been willing to share their personal stories here, often for the first time.*

# Table of Contents

Preface

Choosing Motherhood            11

    The Finest Quality DNA Money Could Buy (by Zoë Sehn)
    Not the Traditional Family (by Shauna)
    Only Regret Is Not Starting Sooner (by Laura F.)
    Meant to Be (by Chelsea)
    This Is the Right Choice (by Megan)

Overcoming Challenges: The journey            35

    Listen to Your Heart (by Samia)
    One Child, Many Blessings (by Marija)
    Twins! (by Laura W.)

The Village That Raises the Child            53

    Beyond Stereotypes (by Rochelle)
    Setting up My Safety Net (by Mali)
    The Craziness Is Made up for by the Love (by Katie W. )
    A Heart Full of Love (by Annie)

Pandemic Parenting     75

    Just Us: Our Little Family of Three in a Pandemic (by Katie Gregory)

    All You Really Need is Love (by Kristi)

Reflections on Parenting     87

    Arrival (by Nadia Pestrak)

    Crazy or Brave? Single and Trying for a Second Child (by Athena Reich)

    Finding My Power in Motherhood (by Myriam Steinberg)

Resource List     108

# Preface

This book was inspired by my own journey to being a choice parent.

When I first thought of having a child on my own, I wanted to learn from those who were already choice parents. I talked to everyone I could think of – friends, acquaintances, people I met at parties – looking for examples of other people who had successfully had children on their own. I had phone conversations with them and asked all sorts of questions. How did you become a parent? Do you ever regret your decision? What have been the hardest moments?

I often wished for more stories, more examples. I wanted to hear multiple versions of what might eventually did become my own future. This anthology is intended as a gift to others who, like my past self, are looking for stories that explore the journey to choice parenthood.

For the purposes of this anthology, choice parenthood is consciously choosing to become a parent without a partner or co-parent. A few of the stories in this volume slightly stretch this definition – suggesting that our definitions need to be as individual as the persons involved.

Many who read this anthology may themselves be considering choice parenthood, or are actively on the journey to choice parenthood. Like me, you may be looking for stories to inspire and inform your own next steps. I hope that these tales of parenthood will help all of us to better understand and appreciate the possibilities in our own futures.

Choice parenthood is not for everyone. Each of these stories is from a person who considered their options and continued on their choice parenting journey. There are many other tales. This anthology does not include stories of those who chose to stay with a partner they loved, even if it meant never having a child; those who tried one or several times, said goodbye to angel babies, and decided not to try further; and those who considered but decided against choice parenting.

The significance of these stories is that each represents a choice – a choice that is not generally expected by society, a choice that was sometimes costly. Whatever your journey, whatever choices you have made and will make, I hope you are inspired by the strength and determination of the parents in this book.

These stories came in response to a call-out for stories from choice parents in Canada through related Facebook groups, as shared in the resource list at the end of this anthology. While this anthology includes a wide range of stories and experiences, it does not represent the full diversity of choice parents. It is my hope that future anthologies, perhaps with a broader geographical scope, might include stories with more gender, socio-economic, and racial diversity.

The anthology has five parts. Becoming a Parent: The Journey shares stories of the journey from decision-making and fertility to finally becoming a parent. Next are a shorter set of stories of Overcoming Challenges – pithy summaries of major life experiences and events leading ultimately to parenthood. The Village That Raises the Child explores ways that choice parents have intentionally cultivated communities of support around themselves throughout the journey to parenthood.

Pandemic Parenting shares stories that delve a little more deeply into the journey of parenting during the COVID-19 pandemic of 2020–21, when established support networks were suddenly removed. The final section contains Reflections on Parenting, with thoughtful and beautiful writing from several parents by choice.

I was moved to tears many times as I read and re-read these stories. I am so thankful to those who gave time and energy to share their unique perspective.

Whatever your path, I hope you are inspired, challenged, and awed by these stories as much as I was.

*Mali Bain*
*Nanaimo, BC*
*November 2021*

SINGLE MOTHERS BY CHOICE

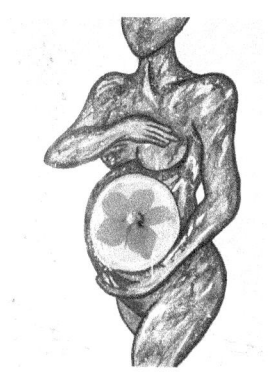

# CHOOSING MOTHERHOOD

# The Finest Quality DNA Money Could Buy

*By Zoë Sehn*

*Zoë lives with her family in the beautiful Okanagan Valley in BC, Canada where she pretends to be an adult, but only until nap time is over. She is a storyteller, tea drinker, blanket fort builder, dreamer, and Mama Bear.*

Growing up, I knew I wanted to become a mother but ordering frozen sperm samples from an online catalogue is not how I imagined I'd start my family. No little girl dreams of becoming a mother to what will begin, essentially, as a popsicle. And let me tell you, all romance ends when someone pulls out a speculum.

I made a deal with myself about motherhood when I decided to complete a PhD. On the cusp of turning 30, I had previously expected that by that point I'd be married with children. I wasn't. Instead, I decided to go back to university halfway around the world in Scotland. With no relationship in sight, I revised my timeline believing that with five years until my mid-30s, I could still live out the stereotypical Rom-Com: have a delightfully quirky meet-cute, fall in love, and get married. There was still lots of time to have babies and, if I was really lucky, they would end up with adorable Scottish accents. The flip side of my deal with myself, however, was that if this little fantasy didn't pan out, God forbid, and I didn't find someone with whom I'd like to combine DNA, then I'd need to use some ingenuity and come up with a backup plan.

I almost got the storybook ending… but not quite.

At 32 I met a man. At 33 we were engaged. At 34 I was blessedly single once more. And by 35? I was just as far from being a mother as I had been at 30, only five years older and $60,000 more in debt. So, I gave myself until I turned 36. Then 37. It was then that I took my motherhood into my own hands and connected with a fertility clinic.

I actually had multiple male friends offer to donate sperm. Some of these offers were made in jest as sexual innuendo. Others were by single friends who saw me as the womb they didn't have. But if I was going to have a child without a husband, I couldn't sit comfortably with the thought that I would be giving up half my parental rights with no real benefit. As partners there is, theoretically, the tradeoff of intimacy, mutual support, and love. Having a child with someone I wouldn't be spending my life with felt like being divorced without the marriage. How could we be guaranteed to have the same parenting plan? How would we divide the holidays? What would happen if they found a new Mommy for my child? It felt like more struggle and potential heartache than I could handle.

Although I started the process of trying to conceive at 37, even while I was dating sperm donation had always been the other option. As time moved ever onward and one bad date blended into another, I had begun to get a feel for the idea of doing it on my own. I was quite open about my consideration of this path to motherhood, including with the men who crossed my path. This was usually in response to the oft demonstrated fear of dating a woman in her mid-30s and the concern of being trapped into immediate commitment. Ironically, it was typically glaringly obvious pretty early on that none of these men would meet even the most basic requirements I had for a father figure for my imagined child, and so they had nothing to worry about.

One man I briefly dated accused me of being selfish when I discussed using a sperm donor for insemination. I actually don't think he was altogether wrong. I was talking about following my dream of motherhood, for me. But to him, the idea of my being a single mother by choice was an affront to men everywhere. He found it unsettling that not only was I talking about having a child on my own, I was actually considering choosing to have a child without a man. Or perhaps more importantly, without him. The story had flipped from him having to hold the desperate 30-something woman at bay and protect his 'testicular assets' to one where these assets were not wanted nor were they needed. It bothered him to such a degree that even when it was obvious we would never work as a couple, he tried to dissuade me by shaming me for even considering becoming a single mother. It was quite dramatic.

The response from others with whom I shared that I was considering becoming a single mother was varied. One couple offered the husband's sperm without hesitation. This posed the unique challenge of trying to gracefully decline and yet preserve the friendship. Other apparently happily married women friends seemed concerned that I was going to try to sleep with their husbands; as if the expanding waistlines and receding hairlines they complained about over coffee somehow had been transformed into Adonis desirability simply as a result of my wanting to have a child. Some people found my decision deeply uncomfortable while others were profoundly supportive.

I didn't go after any friends' husbands and I didn't accept any offers to help with the process. Instead, I chose the finest quality DNA money could buy and now I have a headstrong little comedian, a tiny version of myself. I do sometimes feel lonely when we reach a milestone, or at 3 am when she's teething and I'd give anything for a few hours of undisturbed sleep. However, though it may fall a little more heavily on my shoulders, marital status doesn't change the basic challenges that come with raising a child. And even my PhD doesn't help me wrangle a diaper onto a baby who has decided she'd rather be naked.

No, I never imagined I would be doing this alone but I wouldn't change how she came into the world. Motherhood to me is teaching my daughter by example to reach for her dreams.

# Not the Traditional Family

*Shauna lives in Brampton, Ontario. On top of being a single mom to two amazing kids, She also has two large dogs and four cats. On the rare occasions she gets some free time, you can find her reading or doing crafts.*

My name is Shauna Parsons. I am a 41-year-old single mom by chance to a 24-year-old son and a single mom by choice to a three-year-old daughter. I also have one-year-old identical twin grandsons. I guess my family isn't what you would call the traditional family.

I had my son at seventeen. I was fourteen when I met his father, three years my senior. I thought he was the love of my life. For the four years that I was with him, I was insecure, naïve, and extremely gullible. He knew just how to say things to hurt me and make me feel horrible about myself. He was mostly abusive in an emotional way, but he would get physical at times as well. About six months before I got pregnant with my son, I told him that I thought I was pregnant. He punched me twice in the stomach with all his force. I'm pretty sure I had an early miscarriage, although I didn't tell anyone.

I smartened up when I was eighteen, just after my son's first birthday, but the damage had already been done. Either too disgusted with my body after everything he had said to me over the years, or too afraid of being hurt again, I have pretty much been single ever since. This put a huge damper on my plans for a large family.

As I was getting close to 30, I realized that this was not going to happen. I was running out of time. My dream of a house full of children was lost, but I was desperately hoping to have at least one more. I started considering doing it on my own. As a supply Educational Assistant, I didn't have any job security, my pay wasn't great, and my son and I lived in the basement of my mother's house, but it was a thought that kept creeping into my head.

My family was supportive of my decision. My mom even offered to pay the donor fees if I still wanted to go through with it, once I was settled in my job. Unfortunately, she got diagnosed with stage four lung cancer a few years later. She succumbed to the disease in 2014. About three weeks before she passed away, I was offered a permanent position at a great school not far from my house. I had already been looking at donor websites and doing as much research as I possibly could on using donor sperm. Losing my mom pushed me to get more serious about it. I was now 35 and didn't want to wait any longer.

I was so excited for my first try, but that two-week wait was hell. When I got the call that my result was negative, I wasn't too shocked: I wasn't exactly healthy so I had kind of expected it. I immediately started looking into donors again. I had started keeping track in a binder and made pages of all the donors that I liked, including their pictures and basic info. I also kept track of all appointments and what was said at each of them. I think doing this helped keep me sane throughout the process. I also now have a book detailing my journey that I can show to my child when she's older.

The next month I had my second IUI (intrauterine insemination), this time with my absolute favourite donor who hadn't been available last round. Alas, this attempt resulted in yet another negative, as did the next. I was getting extremely disheartened. Each month getting my hopes up and being let down was really starting to wear on me. I already had depression and anxiety. I managed them pretty well, but this was draining. I was also running out of money.

My doctor suggested taking a bit of time off and explained to me that I might have more luck if I lost 30 to 40 pounds. This broke my heart, but I knew that he was probably right. I ended up taking a little over a year off from trying because, even though I was able to lose almost 50 pounds, I no longer had the money required for more tries.

After we sold my mom's house in 2016, I was able to jump back into my journey, though my first try after the hiatus was negative. I wasn't giving up. The donor that I chose for my fifth cycle was one that I'd had on my list since the beginning. He didn't stand out quite as much as some of the others, but his essay was well written, made him sound smart and adventurous, and ended with the quote, "You are the result of 3.8 billion years of evolutionary success: act like it." I really liked this. It made me think that he had a bit of a sarcastic sense of humour which I am drawn to.

Five tries and almost $10,000 later, I got the call I'd been waiting for: I was pregnant!

I work in a middle school, and at the time my sister worked there as well. My sister and her wife were just getting started on their fertility journey, and she had been my biggest supporter through it all. I went straight to my sister's classroom and broke down after telling her the news.

The nurse who called me said my HCG number was pretty low. She said what matters is that the number doubles, the way it's supposed to. Two days later I had blood work again. My number doubled, but barely. They wanted me to come in again in a week for another test. I was terrified that something was wrong. After this last test, they said my numbers were looking much better and booked my six-week ultrasound. That wait was the worst, but the ultrasound confirmed that I had a healthy, well-placed pregnancy. I was ecstatic; I could breathe again.

Now I had been pregnant before, but it had been 20 years prior, so this felt fairly new to me. I didn't remember all the things I was supposed to feel. This whole pregnancy was pretty uneventful. People kept telling me that I was lucky to have no symptoms, or that they were jealous of me, but I saw it as a curse. I kept thinking it was too easy, maybe I wasn't pregnant anymore, maybe I'd lost the baby, and if I didn't have any symptoms then maybe it wasn't real. I lived for doctor's appointments. Ultrasounds were my favourite thing at this point. They showed me that my baby was real, my baby was okay.

I told my dad and my brother on Father's Day. They knew how badly I had wanted more children and they were completely accepting of my choice to do it alone. Once I'd told my immediate family, I filled in the rest of family and close friends before posting on Facebook. I was a little nervous about this. I had heard stories of others in my situation who didn't have support or who had to deal with rude and hurtful comments about their choice. I didn't have any of this: everyone in my life has been extremely supportive of me and my choice to go this alone.

I found out at eighteen weeks that I was having a little girl, and I actually cried. I was sure I was having a boy. Not only did I not know anything about raising a little girl, but this world is so cruel to girls. I grew up so insecure and so ashamed of my body, and I didn't know how to protect my little one from these feelings. I talked to a dietician and social worker and they were able to assuage my fears a little. It didn't take long for me to start getting excited about having a girl. Let's be honest: clothing and accessories for little girls are so much cuter than those for little boys.

My daughter is now three, and she's a real firecracker. She is the sweetest, funniest, kindest, bravest, most curious girl I have ever met. I wouldn't change her for the world. She's a lot of work at times as she's got her grandma's stubbornness and strong will, as well as her adorable gapped front teeth. She definitely keeps me on my toes.

When my daughter was born, my son really stepped up. He drove me to appointments, he would help out if I needed a break and would babysit so I could get out every once in a while. My son and his girlfriend had twins in September 2019. And when COVID-19 hit in early 2020, my son moved out to be with her and the boys full-time.

This brought out some fears I didn't know I had. I realized that now it was just my daughter and me. What if something happens to her? What if something happens to me? What if I die in my sleep and she's left to cry all alone? This last one is actually my biggest fear: I think about it more than I'd like to. I can handle being a single mom, I can handle the bills, and the boo-boos, and the questions, and the learning and the teaching, but I worry sometimes about being the only parent she has.

I have a great family and know she will be very well cared for, so I at least take some peace in that. I also worry sometimes that she might resent me for not having a dad. I'm completely honest with her about her story. Though young, she understands the basics of it.

Through a Facebook group for people who had used Xytex donors, I found a family who had two children from the same donor, and they connected me to more. I am in contact with nine of my daughter's 'diblings' and know of at least three more. I love watching these children grow and seeing similarities to my daughter. They're all fairly close in age, and I would love for them to be able to meet one day.

The last few years have been a whirlwind of emotions, and being a single mom definitely comes with its challenges, but because of this process I have the most beautiful little girl, and I am at peace with my choice. I no longer long for the house full of kids; I got the one that is perfect for me, and I'm good with that.

# Only Regret Is Not Starting Sooner

*Laura is an Educational Assistant living in Southern Ontario with her daughter, Magnolia. She loves photography, reading, crafting, and especially going on adventures with Noli. Laura hopes to someday add more children to her family and maybe even find Mr. Right!*

My name is Laura and I live in southern Ontario. I have a two-and-a-half year-old daughter and got pregnant fairly quickly, but my road to becoming a choice mom started many, many years ago.

My relationship history is, well, basically non-existent. I've tried to find "Mr. Right" for some time now, but it just hasn't been in the cards for me to this point. I've done online dating, putting myself out there by joining groups and taking classes, and even been open to being set up, but nothing ever clicked with anyone. Looking back now, I think a lot of my bad luck in finding someone could have had to do with my history of depression and anxiety, and my struggles to feel confident and worthy – I'm working on that though. Even though I've never had a relationship, I always knew I wanted to become a mother. From my early twenties onward I always said that, if I hadn't met someone by the time I was 35, then I'd have a baby on my own. This was out there and this was my plan.

The summer I turned 34, I started thinking about this plan. I knew I had a lifetime to find love, but the time to have a baby was much shorter. I was in a position in my life where all my debt was paid off, I had some money for a down payment for a house, and I had a steady job. I wondered why 35 had to be the magical number; why not start now?

I started researching my options more seriously and joined some Facebook groups for Single Moms By Choice. I had no idea there were so many other women in the same position. While acknowledging that I understood these women all loved their children, I made a post asking if they would have done anything differently? Within a day I had over 140 responses, with the majority saying their only regret was that they didn't start sooner. I had my answer!

I was open about my plans with a few friend groups and my parents and was so lucky to be met with nothing but support. I was slightly unsure of how others would take the news, especially those in the church (I'm a Christian), but everyone was so supportive and happy for me.

I made a self-referral to a fertility clinic. I had my first appointment in October 2017, my first IUI in January (which was unsuccessful), a cancelled IUI in February, and got pregnant with my second IUI in March! Things happened fast.

In December 2017, while I was still deciding on a donor, I met another woman, Jackie, who was on her journey to be a choice mom. We both struggled with anxiety and had connected via Facebook. We started talking and became friends. It turned out that we had both chosen the same donor! She was lucky enough to become pregnant in January 2018. It was really exciting to connect with not only another single mom by choice, but one who was carrying my baby's sibling.

My daughter, Magnolia Lucy Mae, made her arrival on October 31, 2018, five weeks early – but at 7lbs, 7oz I'm sure glad she didn't go to term! Not long after her birth, Jackie and I started seeing posts and hearing from other moms who had also used our donor. These connections just kept coming. We now have a total of eleven families with a total of twelve kids (and one more on the way!) from our donor. We have a pretty close group and chat often, as well as video call. Our kids were all born within a year and a half of each other. It's fascinating to see the similarities in both their looks and personalities as they grow. I feel delighted and blessed to be connected to this amazing group of women.

Now that Noli (what I call her) is getting older, we talk a lot about our unique family. She knows she doesn't have a dad, but has a donor instead, and that it doesn't make our family any less because we are so full of love. I've always been open and honest about this journey with her and other people. I want my daughter to feel proud of where she came from and know how truly wanted she was (and is!). I never want her to feel embarrassed or shame because she isn't from a "traditional" family and love that she gets to experience life, not only with me, but her donor siblings.

I am so happy with my decision to become a single mom by choice and I completely agree with those women who had said that their only regret was not starting earlier. It hasn't been an easy job, but it's been the best two and a half years of my life. I am so blessed to be Magnolia's mom. Even though we may not be a traditional family, our love makes it complete.

# Meant to Be

*Chelsea is a first time mom. She lives in Kingston, Ontario and works as a Registered Nurse.*

I spent my twenties with a man who didn't want kids. He told me that when we got together, but at the age of twenty-two this didn't seem like an issue.

Six years later I wanted a family and he still didn't, so we split up. I was devastated. A co-worker suggested that I get pregnant 'by accident' if I really wanted to be with him. I actually considered it for about two seconds, but I knew I couldn't do that to him and it wasn't what I wanted for myself and my future baby. My stepmom is a single mother by choice (SMBC), so when things didn't work out with him, I figured I could always follow in her footsteps if I really had to. I never expected to actually have to do it though!

At the age of 35 I was again dating someone who didn't want kids. Dean had two of his own kids and had had a vasectomy. I decided that I had waited long enough to meet the right guy and started making plans to use a donor. Dean was very supportive of my plans, but still did not want to start another family.

I started trying on my own at the age of 36. Over a two-year period, I was only able to do three intra-uterine inseminations (IUIs) through the clinic with donor sperm because of a combination of the clinic being closed due to COVID-19, regular summer closures, and my miscarriages.

Of my three IUIs, two worked. The first pregnancy was ectopic. It took a few months, three ultrasounds, and over twenty rounds of bloodwork before I was cleared to try again. At the time, I think I was the only woman going for bloodwork hoping that my HCG had dropped. The second attempt failed and the third was another miscarriage. This time, I decided to take Misoprostol to terminate more quickly. I didn't want to wait like I had the first time. I found that drug terrible and I was very sick for a couple days. Still, at least it was over quickly and I could try again.

I had plans for my fourth IUI in March 2020, but my bloodwork didn't look great, so the doctor cancelled my insemination. And then the clinic closed once again because of COVID. At this point I was getting very frustrated and depressed. The miscarriages were not only devastating, but time consuming. I was now 38 years old, the clock was ticking louder and louder every day, and now my baby plans were put on hold for an indeterminate amount of time because of the pandemic.

By the summer of 2020 I couldn't stand the waiting anymore. I found a known donor, had a contract written up, and tried one intra-cervical insemination (ICI) with him. It didn't work. The next month he had a cold and wanted to wait until my next cycle to try again. However, the clinic called and said they were starting to slowly open and could take me. So in September of 2020 I used the sperm that I had had delivered to the clinic the previous December, and it worked!

Dean and I had previously broken up each time I got pregnant. We felt it was best for both of us. However, each time I miscarried we would end up back together. This time we decided to wait and see if I would miscarry again. I didn't, and I gave birth to a beautiful baby boy. I was nervous and unsure about whether or not Dean would actually stay once the baby was born and whether or not we would be able to parent well together. We are still together. He has been amazing and is a fantastic father to our son.

When I was younger, I didn't think I would have to be a SMBC. But once I had decided that was the path I would take, things changed for me. This is not the life I envisioned for myself at any point in my life, but I have never been happier!

# This Is the Right Choice

*Megan is a single parent to an amazing six-year-old! They live in the Greater Toronto Area (GTA) in Ontario and spend as much time outside, exploring nature, as possible.*

I made the decision to become a single mom by choice fairly quickly. However, I did, almost instantly, have a feeling of "Ah yes! THIS was the right choice!"

I always knew that I wanted to be a mom. Having children was extremely important to me. I had conversations with friends over the years where I said, only half seriously, that if I hadn't met the "Right Guy" by the time I was 35, that I would just have a baby on my own.

Fast forward to my 34th year. I had just experienced the worst two and a half years of my life. I had suffered two miscarriages. They truly devastated me. Then my mom got incredibly sick and almost passed away. Thankfully, she pulled through. And then, I discovered my boyfriend, whom I had been trying to have a baby with, was living a double life. He was not at all who I thought he was. It was a really rough time. However, I learned a lot about myself during that time. About how strong and capable I was.

I think that anyone who has ever tried to get pregnant can

probably understand how hard it is to switch that off. When my relationship ended, I still really wanted a baby. I joined some dating sites, but quickly realized that I wasn't looking for a partner. I was looking for a Baby Daddy. I knew that wasn't the story I wanted for my child or for me. It wouldn't be fair to anyone. I had the rest of my life to meet Mr. Right, but my baby-making years would end sooner rather than later.

Shortly before we broke up, my ex and I had been referred to a fertility clinic for recurrent loss testing. They had done all the tests and, other than low AMH for me, everything was fine.

At the time, I knew two different people (a friend and a co-worker) who were going through separations with children involved. One of them (the co-worker) was in a messy break-up, and it got ugly. The children were the ones who suffered the most. The other one (my friend) was in a fairly amicable break-up, both parents were great and loving parents to the child and they were able to maintain a positive co-parenting relationship. But I remember my friend calling me in tears over the Easter weekend. It was the first holiday that she didn't have her daughter with her. She wasn't waking up and experiencing the traditions they had made. It was devastating for her to realize that this would now be the norm for them. My heart broke for her and I couldn't imagine how hard it would be to not have my child with me half the time. To miss out on important events and celebrations. This helped push me to make the final decision.

After talking it over with some close family and friends one weekend, I made an appointment with the fertility doctor. I talked to my mom first and before I even finished explaining my reasons for considering it, she exclaimed, "I think it's a great idea!" She agreed that I needed some time to heal before entering a new relationship, and knew that I would always regret it if I missed my chance to be a mom. I spoke with my cousin and a couple of close friends next, and they all felt the same. It was definitely reassuring to know that I was going into this decision with so much support.

At the appointment, I sat down and said, "He is no longer in the picture. But I still want a baby." She responded, "Well then, let's get you a baby!"

I had first met the fertility doctor when my family doctor referred me for the recurrent pregnancy loss testing. I instantly felt supported and cared for by her. She was extremely thorough and knowledgeable and she genuinely cared. The first time I met her I was filled with a sense of hope that she would help me realize my dream of being a mom. So when I approached her with the information that I would be pursuing parenthood on my own, I had total confidence that she would be supportive.

She was very supportive and excited for me. She helped me navigate the process of choosing a donor and provided a number of resources for me as well. Her support throughout the initial process, and my whole pregnancy, was above and beyond what I could have hoped for. I had a lot of anxiety throughout my pregnancy, because of the past miscarriages, and she helped to reassure me and keep me calm throughout. Weekly ultrasounds and/or heartbeat checks helped immensely. At about twelve and a half weeks I had some bleeding. I called her in a panic and she had me on the ultrasound table within an hour. She had been on her way out of the clinic, but stayed until after my ultrasound to make sure I was ok. She was truly amazing and helped me to be able to enjoy my pregnancy and relax a bit.

After spending a couple of months choosing the "perfect" donor, I started cycle monitoring. I got extremely lucky and got pregnant from my first IUI. My "baby" is about to turn six!

I can honestly say that this is the best decision I have ever made. Not only do I love being a mom, I love being a single mom by choice. People will often comment about how hard it must be to be an only parent. While it definitely comes with challenges that coupled parents may not face, it's also easier in some ways. In the early days after having a baby, you're in a fog. Recovering from childbirth – in my case a traumatic one that ended with me needing a blood transfusion – getting to know your baby, settling into a routine. It takes a lot of energy. I honestly can't imagine having to maintain a relationship at the same time. I felt like I had a bit more freedom to "lose myself" in those early days, because no one else needed my time and attention, so I wasn't letting anyone down.

I also like that I get to parent my way. I get to make the decisions that are right for my daughter and me without worrying about someone else's opinion. I still like the idea of finding my Mr. Right, and I'm sure it will happen someday. But for now, I love the life that my daughter and I have. We are very close and this was definitely the right choice for our family. My daughter is very aware of her story. She will tell people proudly that she has a donor instead of a dad. I have shown her the pictures I have of him and I always answer any questions she may have. One day, out of the blue, she said to me, "Dads are really great, but I'm glad that we have a donor in our family instead of a dad. I think that's better for our family." While this may not be the way I had always envisioned my family, I can honestly say I'm glad this is the way it turned out. I wouldn't change a thing!

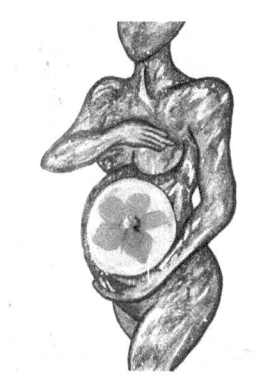

# OVERCOMING CHALLENGES: THE JOURNEY

# Listen to Your Heart

*Samia is a mother of two-year-old twins living in Whidbey, Ontario. She was born into a somewhat conservative Muslim family in Bangladesh.*

Every story of motherhood is unique in itself. Every journey no matter how beautiful is paved with challenges that one cannot always anticipate or prepare for.

I had dreamt of becoming a mother. My soul yearned for the pearls of motherhood. However, my dreams never remotely involved the image of me being a single parent. Dreams are funny that way. We only sketch from what we know. For me, the concept of becoming a single parent by choice was not something I had given much thought to.

To give you a snippet of my past life, I was in a long-term relationship which unfortunately ended. I found solace and comfort in focusing on my career. The busy work life helped me move on. My work achievements made me feel good about myself.

I tried to find time to meet people. While I met many people, there wasn't anyone that I could picture as a true partner; one that I could spend my life with and one that I could have a family with. Both of those had to go hand in hand. I couldn't picture myself being with someone just to have a child. It was simple. If someone couldn't be my true partner, they couldn't be my companion on this journey of parenthood.

My search continued. The days passed by quickly.

I found my 40th birthday knocking on the door.

Opening the door meant opening a flood of questions that gave me anxiety to the point of paralysis. Had I waited too long? Had I forgotten about my biological clock? Should I have considered my options differently? I wanted to have a child, there was no doubt about that. What should I do? What could I do?

My mind first jumped to adoption. As quickly as I could, I tried to educate myself about the processes, paperwork, finances, and most importantly my mental readiness for it. My excitement at the prospect of having a child quickly faded as I learned that adopting a child would be challenging and close to impossible as a single parent.

I spent a few days crying about the unfairness of it all. Why is it not possible to show how much I want to be a mother, and have that be a consideration in the process of adoption? After the tears dried, I realized that as difficult as it would be, I would have to try and become a mother on my own.

Difficult was an understatement. I was almost playing a blind hand at a rigged game where things like my age, my body, my family, my culture, and the life that I had created were all playing against me. I knew there were hurdles that I hadn't even thought of that would be hurled at me along the way.

I started speaking to my friends about this, wondering if someone who was born into a somewhat conservative Muslim family in Bangladesh, could really make my friends and family understand. The words, "This is not socially acceptable" kept flashing in front of my eyes.

My sleepless nights were filled with conversations with my inner fears. A voice would speak out to me, "People will say all sorts of things about you behind your back. They will never understand you". Times like this, I would feel a rush of frustration and would feel myself screaming inside, "Why won't they understand me?!"

There were nights when I lost the fight and went to bed with pillows wet from my tears. But there were nights when my past dreams would come floating in front of me and I could see myself holding a baby close to my heart. I would feel the frustration ooze out of me, to be replaced with tranquility. I would realize that people who loved me and were close to me would try to understand me, and if they couldn't, at least they would support me. There was also a bitter thought at times, when I would tell myself that if someone couldn't do either of the two, maybe I wouldn't want them in my life. My rollercoaster of emotions made sleep very unpredictable.

I finally made my way to some good news. I was pregnant. I was expecting twins. It was such a magical feeling that no matter how much I try, what words I use, how many books I write, I can never fully describe it to anyone. They say it's the best feeling in the world. They say the only way to know it is to experience it. They are right.

I was also overjoyed to know it would be twins. Initially I was nervous when my physician decided that we would transfer two embryos for implantation. At the time, I was told that given my age, having both embryos implant was highly unlikely. Unlikely things happen sometimes. Unlikely surprises can sometimes be good.

My surprise not only made me feel extremely happy about having two babies to love, but it also made me think of life after me. They will always have each other. They will always be there for each other. They will be the best of friends. It was my moment of validation, because I was now certain I had made the right decision. This was extremely helpful to help deal with the next few months.

Did anyone ever tell you that pregnancy takes a toll on your physical body? Well, it really does. Did anyone ever tell you that pregnancy takes a toll on your mental being? Well, it really, really does.

During this crazy journey, I had something else to worry about. I had to now tell the world. More importantly, I had to first tell my family. I was initially cautious in how I approached it but realized that there was no soft way of breaking this news to them. I had to just tell them and make them understand why this was important to me. They were my family; it was important to me that they understood or that I could at least say that I tried my best to make them understand. They were not against the concept, but they were stuck thinking about how they would explain it to other people, what story could justify my actions, and what would be the most acceptable explanation.

There is no better and simpler way to put it – it made me sad. But I realized that it was not their fault, they were brought up and entangled in a society that frowned upon such decisions. They had to find a way to exist in society, while finding a way to understand my decision and the emotions I was going through. I was not ashamed of my decision, because that would mean I was ashamed of my children, which was a blasphemous thought. There was nothing more pure than my children, nothing at all.

It was difficult, but my family and I found our way together. My family understands me. My family loves me. More important than that, my family loves my children, maybe even more than me. They cannot get enough of them. It brings me an element of peace. I have finally learned to trust and lean on those who are close to me. They are here for me emotionally and always here to help. I know I just have to ask.

When you truly want something and work towards it, things often find a way of falling into place. I know there is always an element of luck, destiny, fate, or whatever you want to call it, but you truly have to want something from your heart and work for it. As I see my kids play in front of me, I think back to how things have changed. There is no doubt in my mind, there is no anxiety, frustration or rage.

"Listen to your inner voice. Listen to your heart." As simple as it sounds it is very important. It sounds like something out of a poem, I know. But there is a reason why poems sometimes transcend the borders of culture and community, because they usually stem from human emotions, which are universal. There are certain things that will always hold true, no matter what community you live in, how old you are, what color your skin is, what gender you identify as. This is one of them. Listen to your inner voice. Listen to your heart.

SINGLE MOTHERS BY CHOICE

# One Child, Many Blessings

*Marija is a proud single parent to a wonderful and highly creative child. She resides in Ontario with her daughter and her two cats – Kiwi and Mango.*

Becoming a mom was never in question.

Growing up, I was always fascinated with large families. My father came from a family of nine children. My mother came from a family of five children. John F. Kennedy had three brothers and five sisters. Lucille Ball starred in a movie called Yours, Mine and Ours and they had a total of eighteen children. Steve Martin starred in Cheaper by the Dozen. Yup, you guessed it. They had twelve children.

My dream was to find the right guy, get married, have a career and be a mom to sixteen beautiful kids.

But it never happened. I never fell in love. Oh, I've had my interests and crushes and dated a few guys. But I have never experienced true love.

In the spring of 2007, at the age of 33, I was dating someone that I thought had potential. We had been casual for a while by that time, and I wanted the relationship to progress. However, the signs were there, and I could see that there would be no future with this guy.

Out of nowhere, a thought came to me. Why don't I just start a family by myself? My biological clock was ticking. Fertility is temporary, I thought. As for finding true love and getting married? There is no deadline. It can happen at any age.

I immediately researched fertility clinics near me and called one. However, a referral from my family doctor was required. So I called my family doctor and made an appointment. It was scheduled for my 34th birthday. My doctor was very supportive of my decision. To this day, I am grateful that she was so wonderful.

Shortly afterward, I received a referral for a fertility doctor. The appointment was for four months later. That October day in 2007 I was so excited for my initial consultation. As I got closer to the clinic, a strange feeling came over me. I couldn't help but feel that this was wrong. I shook off my feelings. Maybe I was just nervous?

The consultation went well, and I received a lot of information. All of the procedures and costs were explained to me in detail. However, I still walked out of the clinic with a funny feeling. Maybe this wasn't the right path for me after all. Maybe I was meant to find someone and get married instead.

So I waited.

One year later, in November of 2008, I attended the mandatory appointment with the psychologist at the clinic. This was simply a formality, although I believe it was a government requirement prior to starting the process. The psychologist and I discussed my reasons for wanting to become a single mother by choice (SMBC). I was 35 years old.

Between January 2009 and April 2009, I had several appointments at the clinic involving blood tests to track ovulation, as well as various ultrasounds and other tests.

Still, I did not proceed.

In July of 2009, I was 36 years old. By this time, I had been working as an administrator at a university for ten years. I was preparing to move forward with my plans, but I received a job offer for another administrative position that looked very attractive to me. It was a position that I had been wanting for over a year. I took the job and I put my baby plans on hold.

In late November of 2009, I was doing some planning for the next academic year. I realized that I would soon be turning 37 years old and I was still single. This started to scare me. I had waited so long! I needed to start the process now. The dream job I had was no longer a good enough reason for me to wait.

So I moved forward with my plans. I moved very quickly; I was ready now. It felt right this time.

On January 9th, 2010, I had my first insemination. I did not conceive. Between April and July of 2010, the process of ovulation testing, insemination, and failed attempts happened three more times. I was now 37 years old.

In August I had my fifth insemination. I was tracking my menstrual cycle and I was late. I started to feel hopeful and excited, but unfortunately I experienced some bleeding and very painful cramps. The next day I was bleeding very heavily. I believe that I was pregnant, but that I had lost the baby very, very early. I called the clinic and cancelled the pregnancy test that had been scheduled.

In September, the ovulation period was missed and the insemination could not take place. At this point, I requested fertility drugs in order to speed up the process. I wanted to finally get pregnant! However, the fertility drugs didn't work well for me. And now we were into the month of October.

In November I had my sixth insemination. I had to take progesterone tablets to strengthen my uterus and to help with implantation. About a week later, I experienced stomach cramps. Could this be implantation?! The home pregnancy tests I took all came out positive!! I was pregnant!

Not long after, I went to the clinic for the pregnancy test and was happily waiting for the official results. I found out the test was positive, but the hormone levels were very, very low. That same day, I started feeling some cramps. I became afraid that I was losing the baby. About three weeks after insemination, I began bleeding very heavily and had extremely painful cramps. It was the worst pain I had ever felt in my life. The sixth insemination ended up being a chemical pregnancy, confirmed by the clinic.

By now, I had completed six inseminations and had experienced two chemical pregnancies over a period of ten months.

The seventh insemination was done on January 9th, 2011. This time, I refused to take any home pregnancy tests. I wasn't going to go through all of those emotions again. Feeling somewhat defeated and depressed, I decided that I would keep going until I achieved my dream. When it happens, it happens, I thought to myself.

On January 26th, I took the scheduled pregnancy test at the clinic. And I waited for the call. A few hours later I was told that the pregnancy test was positive. I was not excited. I worried about the hormone levels. It could be another chemical pregnancy. I asked about the hormone levels and the nurse said they looked good. This was for real. I was finally pregnant! The seventh attempt was lucky for me! I felt like I had just won the lottery!

In September of 2011, four and a half years after deciding to become a single mother by choice, I gave birth to a healthy baby girl. She was six pounds and thirteen ounces.

Becoming a single mother by choice was the best decision of my life. The whole process was a roller coaster ride with so many emotions. The biggest emotion I experienced was stress. But what a journey!

I had the pleasure, and the opportunity, to experience a full pregnancy and childbirth. I thoroughly enjoyed these experiences. In my opinion, having a baby is better than having a husband. Marriage can dissolve. But the relationship I have with my daughter is permanent.

When it comes to regrets, I only have one. I wish I had started earlier because I wanted to have more than one child.

But the number of blessings that resulted from this decision are numerous. I may not have the sixteen children that I always dreamed about, but I have so many blessings because of this one child.

# Twins!

*Laura lives in Toronto, Ontario. She is a 47-year-old mom of two-year-old twins. She works full time. She loves Disney and New Kids on the Block (yes the group).*

I'm a single mom by choice with double-donor twins.

My journey started in a coffee shop while talking to friends about wanting to be a mom, with no partner in sight. One of them mentioned using a sperm donor through a fertility clinic. This idea made me feel more positive.

My old-school but encouraging family doctor sent a referral to the fertility clinic, and the journey began. Although I started to have appointments with my first clinic, they wanted me to lose weight and the process was unsuccessful. I moved on to another clinic, where I did three IUIs, but my weight again became an issue, and they wouldn't allow me to do IVF. I spoke to a new family doctor (as my old one retired) and she told me she would find a clinic to help me. Well, she did.

I moved on to IVF and had a total of three retrievals. I was able to get pregnant, but never stayed pregnant past twelve weeks. I started looking into using an egg donor. I knew it wasn't the sperm, as I had tried different donors, so I concluded that it must be my eggs.

I did lots of research on my own. I looked into embryo adoption, egg donation and surrogacy. I ruled out surrogacy because I wanted to try to carry my child. I actually approached my fertility doctor with the idea of using an egg donor and we talked about it. He gave me his professional medical advice and we were both happy with my choice to move to donor eggs. It was a very easy choice for me.

In September 2018, my donor had her retrieval. There were 52 eggs retrieved, and a total of eighteen made it to day 5/6. All were high grade. I was super excited. There was hope. I had all these chances to make my dreams come true.

During the lead up to transfer day, my doctor and I talked about how many embryos to transfer. He wanted one, but I wanted two. He knew of my struggles to remain pregnant, so he agreed to two. Even though I'm an identical twin myself, we shook hands on agreeing not to have twins.

Six days past the five-day transfer, I took a home pregnancy test and it came up positive. But I had been through this before and didn't want to get too excited. I phoned my clinic to book an earlier blood draw, went in at eight days past the transfer, and the test came back positive at 364hcg. I was so happy. My dreams of becoming a mom finally seemed possible.

At my five-week ultrasound I found out I was having twins. In spite of my earlier agreement with the doctor, and even though I knew there was still a long road ahead to having healthy babies, I was actually super happy to hear this. I did what I could to look after myself. At 20 weeks I found out I was having a boy and a girl. This was even more special, as my son is the first boy in our family in 52 years.

I had my children via a scheduled C-section at 36 weeks and

five days. They were perfect! Twenty little fingers, twenty little toes, cute little faces. I knew these were the babies I was meant to get.

Through all my struggles, I remained positive knowing they would come to me when the time was right. Thankfully, I live with my twin sister and her daughter, who are a huge help. I wouldn't have my life any other way. When they call me mommy, or run to me when they're hurt or sad, it proves to me that, genetically or not, they're mine, all mine! I built those bodies, nourished them, grew them, and I love them with my whole being.

SINGLE MOTHERS BY CHOICE

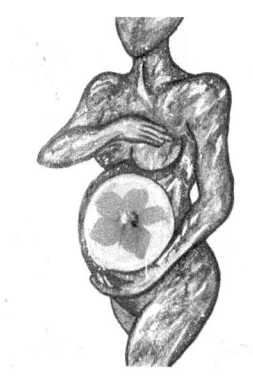

# THE VILLAGE THAT RAISES THE CHILD

# Beyond Stereotypes

*Rochelle is a public servant and community organizer residing in Ontario. Her personal time is spent engaging and developing anti-racism strategies for her local municipality, rollerblading, and advocating for the deaf community.*

I first considered becoming a single mom by choice at 28. I vaguely remember having a discussion with my gyno and being referred to a reproductive endocrinologist (RE). At the time, I was not given many resources but just a referral. I wasn't ready then, so I put it on pause.

It wasn't until I experienced another failed relationship and a broken engagement that I decided it was time to explore my options. Honestly, I held back at first because I really wanted to find a life partner to raise a child with. I grew up in a loving home with two parents, and a particularly amazing father. I felt like I would be putting my child at a disadvantage by him not having two parents. I also didn't want to be considered your stereotypical single black mom. Although this was a choice, the potential social rejections and assumptions weighed heavy.

Thankfully I was in a good position emotionally and financially. I made the leap that I would be committed to my journey of motherhood independently.

When I started trying, I set my expectations extremely low. I was in many single mothers by choice tryer groups and witnessed a lot of heartbreak. According to my research, at best I had a 15% chance of it working the first time. I went in thinking it wouldn't work and did my best to remove the emotional aspects of it failing. One of the hardest aspects was grieving not having a partner to go on this journey with.

I had always wanted to be a younger mom. So I took my chances at 31, met with my RE and guess what? My 15% chance became a reality on the first try. I was 100% fearful, but grateful to be in a position that I would soon be a mom. Better yet, this wonderful news was confirmed on my 32nd birthday. Things were starting to come full circle.

The day I had my IUI, the first case of COVID-19 appeared in Canada. Much of the two-week wait was consumed with the unknowns of COVID-19. We were scrambling at work, trying to assess the impact COVID-19 would have on our events. Work kept me going during that wait.

Due to the effects of COVID-19, I had no support at the beginning when it came to attending doctors appointments. Protocols had also changed at my obstetrician's office, leaving me anxious that I may not be getting appropriate care due to COVID-19 restrictions. I was also faced with the fact that I may have to give birth alone. Eventually things got better as restrictions were lifted.

Thankfully, by the time of my son's birth, my sister was able to be my birthing partner. My dad helped me with getting groceries, and my mother took on night shifts so I could rest. My tribe was in full force and supportive. Emotionally, I turned to SMBC and mommy-to-be forums to prepare myself for the next steps into motherhood.

My son is biracial (Caucasian and Afro-Caribbean). I currently live in a predominantly white neighbourhood. I had fears that he may have difficulty with his identity and integrating comfortably within the neighbourhood as he grows because we look different from one another. I have come to realize that the asetethics of our skin colour are no barrier to our bond. I have made steps to actively participate in anti-racism committees within the municipality, so that as he grows within our community, he won't face racial barriers. I am confident that while raising him, he will be proud of his cultural identity, while the neighbourhood slowly becomes multicultural.

Another obstacle to overcome while raising my son has been his potential feelings. He may assume he was abandoned by his biological father, or he may believe that my decision was selfish. I am making it a priority to ensure he is culturally informed about both sides of his heritage and conception, early and consistently as he grows. It's important to emphasize that he is loved and very much wanted by those in our community/tribe.

I have been in contact with three moms of my son's donor siblings. I feel exceptionally lucky that the parents of my child's siblings have been forthcoming and welcoming. I think it's important to foster these relationships. As parents, we can teach our children that knowing their biological ties is their right and should not be denied. It's important for our children to have access to this information and know who they are so that when ready, our children can connect. In a few years I also plan to give him complete DNA testing to confirm his ancestry. I want to be able to provide him as much context as possible about his biological make up and family tree.

# Setting up My Safety Net

*Mali is a single parent living on Snuneymuxw territory (Nanaimo) in British Columbia. She is the owner of NextGen Story: Custom Publishing and parent to a loveable two-year-old.*

I have always looked for ways to live in community settings, and loved working with and teaching children. But it took a significant head injury for me to finally starting thinking about having my own child.

One February evening I went night-skiing for the first time on Cypress Mountain. I had become accustomed to downhill skiis, but this was one of my first times trying out cross-country skiing. It was a crisp minus one degree Celsius, and the surface snow that had melted during the day had frozen into glistening ice. After going up and up for the first thirty minutes or so, we had our first glorious downhill stretch. I put my skis into the classic ski grooves and tucked to get some speed, thinking I'd coast to the bottom of the first hill and up the next one. When the grooves ended, I tried to slow down with the usual "snow plow" manoeuvre – but my skis stopped and I kept going. I went from a vertical position to a horizontal one far, far too quickly.

The next morning, I couldn't get out of bed. Over the next

weeks and months, as I dealt with dizziness, headaches, and complete overwhelm, I was in denial about my concussion. When I did eventually seek help, the (erroneous) medical advice I received was to stay still and do very little - "be in a dark room, bored". Prior to the accident I had a very full life, but by June of 2017 I was struggling to even walk a few blocks from my house.

In the depths of depression one day, I spoke to my sister to lament that I now felt that I would never have a family. I was 37 years old, single, and not even dating. How would I ever meet a partner, get to know them, and have a family?

She said, "Well, you could have a baby on your own – I know people who have done that."

I dismissed the idea, thinking I could never have a child without a partner. Parenting seemed like so much work even for two people. I couldn't imagine doing it on my own.

But the seed had been planted. The next day I called her back and asked, "Could I talk to the people you know?"

I talked to my sister's friends and other friends of friends. I asked about the best parts, the hardest parts, and their regrets. Two themes emerged from those conversations. Many people said something along the lines of, "I don't know why I didn't ask for more help." And, many single parents talked about loneliness in the evenings after their child had gone to bed.

With those insights in mind, the first step for me was setting up shared housing. I found two friends who shared my vision of collective living with a child. We rented a big, beautiful house with three kitchens, four bathrooms, and room for six adults (and one child).

Just over a year later, as I continued to recover from the concussion, I started trying to conceive. After five unsuccessful IUIs and an IVF orientation, I decided to do one more "bonus try" of IUI. I found out I was pregnant just before Christmas, one year and eleven months after my concussion.

In early January, I went on a solo retreat to reflect on the life that I wanted to create for my baby and me. A big theme that emerged was community. As a choice mom once put it, my job as a choice mom is "to convene the village that raises the child."

I decided to host a gathering. I called it "a Celebration of Aunties, Uncles, and Other Such Relations". I booked three group campsites and invited people whom I saw as a part of my extended friend-family. It was such a joy to gather so many friends in one place. Two friends hosted a beautiful ritual for me, which allowed my friends to share their good wishes and also had me step, symbolically and literally, into a new space of actually asking for help.

After this celebration, I reflected on the advice of other choice moms and my own experience and realized that I was unlikely to ask for help when I would need it most. I would need to set up a safety net in advance and then be able to cancel or reduce my supports if I found that I did not actually need the help.

Over the next months, I connected with and hired an amazing post-natal doula. I set up a helping website through lotsahelpinghands.com and listed shifts of 'baby time,' meal train, help with errands, etc. I sent out a mass email to my community in early August, just under a month before my due date. I waited a whole week without anyone signing up.

I remember having the feeling that my safety net might just have some pretty big holes in it. I had sent the email in early August - some people were on holiday, others were busy, but eventually people did figure out the website and sign up to help.

The amazing thing is that somehow, when my daughter was born, it all worked out beautifully. My daughter was birthed into a circle of women. A dear friend came and stayed with me for two weeks and my roommates each helped out in their own way. I was so fortunate in many ways: my midwives were amazing, my friends helped in all the ways they could, and I was just in the flow of doing all these new things required to keep my little one alive. I had many challenges those first few months, but I didn't once feel an absence of support from my community.

Six months later in February 2020, my daughter and I were in Kenya for six weeks visiting my sister and her family. Two weeks before our outbound flight, the first COVID-19 case was declared in Kenya. Four days later, the Government of Canada issued a warning that all Canadians should return home while commercial flights were still available. After several hours on hold with the airline, I was lucky to book a flight home on what ended up being the last KLM flight out of Nairobi.

At the time the Canadian government required all returning travellers to "self-isolate" for fourteen days after entering Canada. And so my daughter and I returned to our collective home to find a new plastic wall in the house, MacGyvered out of plastic sheeting and packing tape. My daughter and I had a kitchen, bathroom, bedroom, and outside entrance. We were to spend fourteen days completely and utterly on our own.

We had groceries dropped off and some food in the freezer (thankfully, left over from the generous meal trains post-birth). I did take her out for walks in the carrier, staying well away from any other pedestrians and not entering any shops or buildings, but apart from that, it was just us: no roommates, no friends, no community.

In retrospect I can see that through those days came a deep

realization that we would be okay, just my daughter and I. Just like the concussion, the quarantine stripped me of the events, activities, projects, and relationships that seemed to give life meaning. Even without all those things, I realized that I could keep going and that our lives had value, just as simple as they were. Life is a lot better with our safety net close by: but we can make it on our own, she and I.

Since then, my life has unfolded and changed in ways that I could never have imagined. What hasn't changed is the certainty of my decision to have a child and the joy I get from the simple life that she and I are so fortunate to live.

# The Craziness Is Made up for by the Love

*Katie W. is a solo parent to a precocious four-year-old and co-foster parent/aunt to her nine-year-old nephew and fifteen-year-old niece in Dundas, Ontario. Currently on a PhD break due to COVID-19, she has created a small business making educational busy bags for young children.*

I became interested in becoming a single mom by choice because of my niece, whom I have been co-raising since she was born. My sister has an intellectual disability, mental health and addiction issues. She's not capable of parenting alone without what we call "the village". So when my niece was born, I was very involved in her life. I had her every other weekend, even when I was away at university. She would come and stay at my apartment. When I moved to Ottawa to do my PhD, she would come and stay with me for a full week every month. So she was always with me.

I had always wanted children of my own. In high school I volunteered to take the electronic baby home over a long weekend. I have been babysitting since I was twelve.

I was interested in having my own child in part because of the relationship I had with my niece, and in part because I had absolutely no control over how she was being raised. Depending on my sister's mood and who she was dating, she could, and did, block us from seeing my niece, and later my nephew. I felt like I had spent all this time and energy raising other people's children without getting to be a parent, and getting to raise a child the way I believed was best. With my niece I had a connection, but not the rights that go along with it. So, it was in part a sort of "control freak" thing and in part just because I loved her so much. I wanted to have that with my own kids.

When I moved to Ottawa for my PhD, I had just gotten out of a long-term relationship. I'm gay, and I was always going to have kids with a sperm donor or in some other "non-traditional" way. So it wasn't a big leap for me to start the process alone. The person I had been with was significantly younger than me and wasn't interested in starting a family yet. But talking about it with them had got me thinking. Since I was doing my PhD and was going to be fairly independent after the first year, as far as my timeline/work schedule goes, I thought it was a really good time to have a child.

The timing all worked out really well. By the time I got all of the stuff pulled together, I had finished my classes, and on my third IUI I knocked myself up. I finished my comps, which is the second part of the PhD, basically two big essays, the month before I gave birth.

Four months after I had my son, my sister stopped being able to care for her kids full time, and her two kids moved in with me and my mom. My mother and I were sharing a rental house and she was supposed to only be there part time, because she lived up north with my stepfather. However, it ended up with everybody living there full time with my four month old and me. That was a smidge challenging!

My son never slept. He had acid reflux, so he had to be held upright when he was sleeping. My aunt would come over every week and just sleep in a chair with him, or I would sleep in a chair with him during his naps. Even when I got him on meds and he was doing better he didn't sleep well. I didn't really sleep for longer than five hours in a row, often no more than six hours in a 24-hour period, for almost a year. All that combined with C-section recovery, breastfeeding issues, and going from being a single person with cats to a mother in a multi-generational household with three (or sometimes four) other people was a lot to deal with.

The first few years were really hard. Everybody was adjusting. Just before my son turned one, we moved again into a bigger house because the kids were staying with us permanently. Then, my mom had knee replacement surgery a month after that move. So she was laid up in bed recovering from surgery. Through all of this, I just plowed forward. You have to, right? That's what single parenthood is. You just have to keep going. There is nobody else.

My kiddo is awesome. He's suspected gifted, which comes with a lot of high needs and quirks. Just watching him learn and figure out new things is amazing. He has just started doing this thing where he will be playing or walking around and will stop and just be like, "Mom? I love you." All the craziness gets made up for by the love. There are the good moments, there are the bad moments, there are the "Oh my God, I'm gonna tear my hair out, I need to go hide in the kitchen for five minutes!" moments, but it's all good.

To those considering being a choice parent, I would say that you cannot under-stress the importance of a village. Yes, you can do it all on your own because you have to. But any kind of support system, any kind of help, even if it's paid help, can take a bit of the load off so that you're not having to do every single thing by yourself. It's just so important. For me, a lot of it is family. I'm lucky that way. My mom can help out occasionally. My niece was eleven when my son was born, so she's fourteen now, and they love to hang out. It's good to see the relationship between them. And then I have friends from childhood, university, and college – people who stuck. With the pandemic everyone has to isolate and look to their own families right now. So we don't see a lot of them, but even just being able to call to commiserate helps. Having someone to share the stories with also helps.

I have ADHD. It's just another layer. In one way, it's kind of helpful because ADHD people are good in a crisis. We're better in a crisis than we are in day-to-day life. I have a hard time doing my dishes but stick me in a crisis, and I am great. My ability to kind of roll with the punches is heightened. I think it would be more difficult for a neurotypical person to go through my life the way that it's been. With the kids, and the changes, the moves, and all that stuff my life basically is a crisis.

But in some ways, it's really, really challenging because I get bored very easily. So, when you're sitting there with a kid who wants to play the same game over and over again, it can make you want to pull your hair out. I know that's probably challenging for literally everybody, but I am bored half-way through game one. So I'm looking at my phone, or sorting something out, or knitting when we play a game. Knitting is the best one to do because I'm not looking at a phone or seeming distracted. I can pay attention to my child, but I'm still doing something. You just kind of have to find coping techniques.

The only other thing that I have learned since having my son has to do with the community of children/people/adults born from donor sperm, and the ethics of being involved with clinics, sperm banks and the lack of laws that regulate it all. By getting involved in Facebook groups I learned how donor-conceived adults feel growing up not having some of the information they might want regarding their genetic family, and how many feel they were robbed of a relationship with the other half of their genetic family. I chose an open ID donor, whom my child can have information on and possibly meet at 18. I knew this was a better choice than being anonymous, which is becoming illegal in many countries worldwide.

I have also connected with my son's donor siblings' parents on Facebook. I would suggest doing this to everybody. My son has a funny toe on his foot that sticks up a bit: definitely not something he gets from my family. I posted it to the group and asked: "Do your kids have these toes?" And I got back all these pictures of other children's feet from somewhere else in the world, and they have the exact same funny toes as my son. All the kids have the same eyes and noses; you can see what the dominant genes are when looking at the group, and it's super neat. But it is also so great for him to have this normalized and available to him.

I hope that having that information as he grows up, and knowing his story from the beginning, will make up (as much as is possible) for me not really understanding the complexity of my decision. Do your research, be open and honest and get involved. Starting right at birth: just tell your kiddo their story.

# A Heart Full of Love

*Annie lives in the Montréal area, in Québec. She is the single mother of an almost two-year-old ray of sunshine! Annie and her son are surrounded by a loving family and great friends.*

I wanted to share my journey, but I found myself completely blocked when trying to write about it. I didn't know how to start, until one word kept coming back in my mind: love.

My "single mother by choice" story is actually a love story – a mother's love to a child she didn't yet have. A child I deeply loved and desired decades before he was even conceived!

When I was a teenager, if you'd ask me how I saw myself "in ten years", whatever answer I would give was only accessory to the fact that I was going to be a mom. I don't think I even mentioned having kids because for me, it just went without saying! I imagined having a typical nuclear family: a husband, a dog, and a white picket fence.

More than ten years had passed and I was nowhere close to that! I eventually got married. My biological clock may have made me rush into that marriage. I couldn't get pregnant and my doctor suggested it might be because I was overweight. The love for the child I was now unable to conceive encouraged me lose over 130 lbs. But then I realized how deeply unhappy I was in my marriage. The only thing that had kept me from ending it was the thought of having a family. And then my husband said that he never even wanted to have children, but didn't want to tell me because he was afraid I would have left him.

The day after my marriage ended, I felt like I could breathe for the first time in years! Within a few weeks he moved out, and I rearranged my home and got my life back on track.

So there I was, at 37, 130lbs lighter but single once again. I looked at my life and realized I had a great job, a very comfortable house, a loving family, and great friends. I was in better shape physically and mentally than I had ever been. I imagined myself ten years down the road. The thought of still being single didn't upset me whatsoever. However, when I thought of not having children, I panicked: an actual anxiety attack! So by that point, the path to take was clear to me. A few days later, I was calling to make an appointment at a fertility clinic.

I was somewhat anxious to talk about my project with my friends and family, but was pleased to receive nothing but support from everyone. My brother and sister-in-law, my friends, my closest colleagues – I was supported and loved all around. I think my mother knew even before I did that this was what I would be doing! Before I even had my first appointment at the clinic, my father was planning how we'd have to install baby gates in the stairs of my home. Love.

So it was with a heart full of love, hope, excitement and anticipation that I started the fertility process. Every blood draw, every uncomfortable ultrasound, every medical exam were only steps bringing me closer to the child I was longing for. I was unbelievably fortunate that my second IUI was the one that would give me the beautiful baby I always loved and hoped for.

At the end of the infamous two-week wait, the fertility clinic I was going to did a blood test. I got the phone call announcing that I was pregnant two days before my 38th birthday. I was having dinner with my family the next day, so I decided to wait until we were all gathered before I told them.

I bought my nephew a t-shirt that said "big cousin", and just in case that wasn't clear enough, I wrote a card from the baby saying he was on the way, with my due date. Everybody went crazy! My mom could barely stand on her feet! As for me, I think I started to fully believe it only after the viability ultrasound (around the 8th week). After I heard the heartbeat and saw all of the activity that was going on in my uterus, I started to fully appreciate what was happening!

I completely understand people choosing to wait until the end of the first trimester before they start telling people. However, being in the close knit family that I am, they pretty much knew everything that was happening and were fully aware of the testing dates, so there was no way I could have hidden it. Plus, I am the absolute worst liar and I figured that if I was to have a miscarriage, I would need them in my corner, so they had to know anyway!

One of the fears I had of being a single mother by choice was that it would be sad or lonely living the pregnancy and the milestones on my own. But I came to realize that I was probably even more surrounded than people in relationships because everyone around me felt involved. Everyone who loved me felt connected to that baby. That tiny little baby growing inside me was loved by so many people even before he was born!

My mom came to every ultrasound. When I got a scare at 23 weeks pregnant, she was with me early in the morning to take me to the hospital. I could see she was just as terrified as I was, waiting to hear the heartbeat on the nurse's monitor. She came to the prenatal classes, breastfeeding workshops, and anything that seemed remotely important to me. She's the one who accompanied me when I gave birth, and now she says that "she delivered this baby!" She spent the first five to six weeks at home with me and my son. Her help and support have been immeasurable.

I am just so unbelievably grateful. And I can't believe how lucky my son is to have so many wonderfully loving people around him, even with the smallest things! I had a co-worker who baked muffins, a friend who brought cases of toys, friends who brought meals, and a friend who called now and then and made sure we talked about things other than baby or motherhood.

"A mother's love." I knew of the expression. I am only starting to comprehend the strength of that love! My son will soon be two years old. I am so ridiculously proud of the tiny human that he is, and of the multitude of things he learns on a daily basis. I had no clue that love could grow so deep it physically hurts. I keep thinking, there is no way I can love him more. But I am wrong. Every, Single, Time!

My love story continues! There are – and will be – many challenges to face. But the love for this child I have waited so long to hold, kiss and hug is helping me get through every one of them.

The first thing I told my son when he was born represents my journey the best: I've been waiting for you for sooooo long.

I am fully aware that my story is far from representative of what some women are going through during their personal journey. But I remember, during a much darker period of my life, feeling like hope for better days was the candle lighting my path, and that this candle had been blown out. I am hoping that my story could be a kindle to re-light someone else's blown-out candle. There are better days to come.

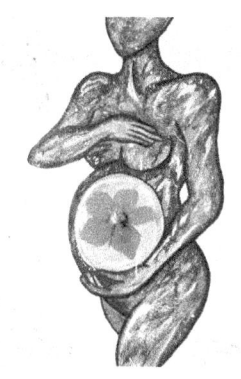

# PANDEMIC PARENTING

# Just Us: Our little family of three in a pandemic

*By Katie Gregory*

*Katie is a single parent of two energetic kids aged three and one year old. She lives in Waterloo, Ontario. She is an infectious diseases physician at a large community teaching hospital.*

I never thought I would need a plan B to motherhood.

I met my now ex-husband when I was seventeen. Just prior to my eighteenth birthday we started dating. We had much in common, including future goals for career and kids, as well as many common interests. In fact, we met volunteering together, doing first aid at a hockey game, which happened to be two of those shared interests. Fast forward to thirteen years later, and our marriage ended. With age, my ex discovered he did not want to have children and I realized that no matter how much I loved my partner, I needed to have children.

The last few years of our marriage saw him trying to figure out for sure that he did not want children. When he finally was confident, I wasted no time. I proceeded to seek out fertility assistance with the help of a sperm donor and a reproductive endocrinologist and got pregnant on my first medicated intrauterine insemination.

I had my daughter in 2018 in the city I used to live in, which was about 75 minutes from my new home. We went home when she was three days old. Three ladies and a baby: three ladies being my mother, my sister and myself. My mom stayed with me for two weeks and then it was us. Just us. Just my perfect little girl and me.

I work primarily as an infectious diseases (ID) physician and do a few nights per month working as an intensive care physician. My daughter and I found a great rhythm when I returned to work when she was nine months old.

I got pregnant with my second in 2019 and had a due date in early March 2020.

I still remember the first time I heard about COVID-19. It was in a group for female infectious diseases physicians. I also still have the first local public health "Alert notice" to physicians pinned on my bulletin board at work. Over the years there have been some different scares as an ID physician, and admittedly back in mid-January I was really not worried. By late January I was having weekly meetings on COVID-19 and feeling a bit odd about both having a baby in what might turn out to be a pandemic, as well as thoughts on how I might feel being an ID doctor on maternity leave during a pandemic.

My son decided he did not want to be in hospital during all that and showed up a month early. During labour I wrote some necessary emails. Postpartum day one or two, a colleague came to my room and I gave handover on my patients. After about a week in hospital, my late preterm baby was able to come home.

This time both my parents came for two weeks to stay with us, and my daughter stayed in daycare. Not having to do the drive to daycare was a huge help. Trying to figure out breastfeeding with my toddler in care was also a help. My son never really got great at the whole nursing thing. I was blessed with lots of milk supply early on, so with a mix of pumping and nursing he was well fed. Talks of a pandemic continued to worsen and then, of course, as you all know, it became very much a reality.

My daughter got sent home for illness (not COVID-19) on a Thursday, and then the next day the daycare was closed indefinitely. My newborn was five weeks old. He was not sleeping well, and I had finally broken down the week prior and hired a night nanny for a couple nights per week. Then suddenly it was "Just Us" in much more real a way than it had ever been before. Our little family of three. It was hard. The night nanny was no more and I focused on us surviving each day. My freezer was well stocked, thankfully, so that was one less thing on the to-do list. I made a daily Instagram post for family and friends. It was entitled "Gregory Physical Distancing Day #". It had the good, the bad, and the ugly.

After just over four weeks of just us, I felt like I hit a breaking point. I called one of my closest friends. One I had only met in 2018, when I hosted a 'Single Mothers by Choice' gathering at my home. Our daughters were only a few months apart. We had similar parenting styles and I knew she felt somewhat trapped in the confines of her condo. She was trying to work from home with an almost two-year-old. I asked if she would be willing to move in so we could help each other for a week or two. We were nervous about harming our friendship, with neither one of us having lived with anyone (other than my ex-husband) for fifteen years.

Thankfully, it did work out. We both knew how to give each other space, and actually gave each other breaks. We had three kids aged two and under plus my dog. It was a bit of a mess, but we got through and it gave me some sense of sanity. Once I felt a bit more back on my feet she returned to her own home.

When she left, my son was sleeping a bit better. Since had I gotten some sleep (thanks to her), I had been able to spend some more time figuring out ways to help my son sleep better. Thankfully in late spring/early summer we got to spend some time with my parents thanks to some relaxation of the rules.

In September I returned to intensive care unit (ICU) work and in January to full time ID work. My son had just turned eleven months in January. During the ICU work in the fall my parents babysat my children, my shifts being 5 pm to 9 am. They would stay in the morning to watch my son so I could have a nap. In January my daycare re-opened the infant room just in time to take my son.

My life now is both easier and harder than it was in 2020. I love my job as a physician. I am passionate about helping patients and families. I pride myself on both being a great clinician and on being able to speak in a variety of way to help someone understand their illness and the plan.

I was destined to be a mother, but I was not destined to be a stay-at-home mother. COVID-19 restrictions have been very stressful. My daycare hours are 8 am to 5 pm. It is really challenging to be a physician and get to a daycare pickup prior to 5 pm. Thankfully my brother's children go to the same daycare, so there are days when he has sat with my children in the parking lot and other times when I have had to pay the fees for being late.

Even more challenging have been the absences. My daughter had been to daycare before, so she had few illnesses, but for my son this was his first major exposure to other people. This has resulted in many absent days while awaiting COVID-19 test results, not to mention his fourteen day quarantine when he was exposed to COVID-19 at daycare. All these absences mean I have a moment of panic every time my phone rings, and it rings a lot when I am on call.

Will it be the daycare? If it is the daycare will my kids be excluded from care? Working from home as a physician with two small children under foot is not fun nor is it efficient.

I would most definitely do it all over again. I have always wanted three or four kids and have talked myself into two as a single mother by choice. To have three or more would be challenging to put my all into both parenting and work. I spoke about having my second the day my daughter came home from the hospital and I only doubted the plan on particularly rough pregnancy days. But for all the planning I did do, despite training as an infectious diseases physician and a diploma in tropical medicine and hygiene, I never predicted what it might be like to solo parent two children during a pandemic.

# All You Really Need Is Love

*Kristi is a single parent by choice to a beautiful, spunky and curly haired one-year-old little girl. She has a passion for adventure and traveling the world which she will show her girl. She lives in Grande Prairie, Alberta and loves being a super mom but pays the bills as environmental consultant.*

My journey to become a single mom by choice was not rushed. It all started two years before attempting to conceive. In the past, I had struggled with relationships to find my life partner. I found myself in my forties, and without a committed partner. When I really started thinking about having a family I was dating a guy, and deep down I knew I didn't want to be with him for the rest of my life. Why would I want to have a child with him? So we broke up. The best advice I was given was to start gathering information about becoming a single mom.

So I looked up a clinic and I made an appointment. I continued to date, always in the hopes of finding someone to create a family with. But to no avail.

I had doubts. Would I be able to financially support a child on my own? Would I lose my freedom, possibly lose friends? What challenges would this process add to dating, and what possible limitations would it put on any future travelling?

All this caused me to hesitate. I put the decision on hold, even though the fertility doctor noted that I had limited eggs and advised me not to take too long. But I knew I needed more time to decide what was best for me. On a motorbike trip in Namibia, I decided that I was ready for the next step and that what was missing from my life was a child. So upon my return, I booked back into the clinic.

I never once considered a known donor. I never wanted to share my child. After a long process of analyzing, I picked a donor from a sperm bank. This was not an easy process as there were an overwhelming number of donors available. I had to decide what was important to me, which was medical history, height, education, athletic ability and more. The donor profile had photos as a child and adult, audio recording and letter with his profile.

My conception was fortunate. I rode my motorbike to the clinic in Edmonton and got inseminated that morning. I remember the nerves and anxiety that it was actually happening. I then continued on a motorbike tour in Montana. When I got back I was working in a remote community in British Columbia (eight hours away from my city). I had to go get a blood test at the remote hospital and get the results sent back to Alberta. It was confirmed the day of my friends' wedding that I was pregnant.

I will always remember the phone call. The nurse told me and then there was a long pause. She then said congratulations, and I was silent. Then I repeated to myself, this is really happening.

My pregnancy was standard, with the added extra care and testing because it was considered a geriatric pregnancy. I was forty-one at this point. However, my delivery and the days afterward were far from standard. I chose to have my daughter, but I didn't choose to have her during a pandemic. I was induced for three days (due to my age) and on the night of the third day I went into labour. I had planned to have my mother with me, but she had to finish her quarantine after returning from the United States. So I asked my two close friends to be part of my delivery team. After 25 hours of labour, my baby girl was born.

She was taken to the neonatal intensive care unit (NICU), which is where we spent the next four days. During delivery she had had the cord wrapped around her neck. She had gotten stuck in the birth canal and went into respiratory distress, with a possible infection and fever. I held her for one minute after she was born before she went to the NICU.

The next day the hospital didn't allow visitors and I was discharged under 24 hours. I spent the next four days in the NICU by myself with my girl. Over the next few weeks, I found strength I never knew I had. During the whole process of the fertility clinic and pregnancy I went to all my appointments by myself. I decided that if I chose to have this baby on my own, then I needed to do it on my own. Unknowingly, this prepared me for the next stage of raising a child during a pandemic.

Baby girl and I were on our own. Alberta was going into lockdown and the world was changing. The nurses were scared and nervous. I was a new mom, on my own, in a place where COVID-19 patients were soon to be arriving. The hospital was all prepared.

Baby girl and I were a bit of a novelty. Who was this mystery baby with one older parent? One nice nurse sat down with me, helped me with the baby, and listened to my story. She was so kind and caring. My hormones and anxiety were both high.

The day I left the hospital with my baby girl I thought I had contracted COVID-19. This was neither rational nor logical thinking as there were very few known cases in the area.

My friend dropped off my truck with the baby car-seat at the hospital, and I drove myself home. I spent the next five days on my own with baby. My goal was to keep my baby safe from the world. It was a struggle to get her to breastfeed and latch, a struggle to wake her up every three hours to feed, a struggle to feed myself, and a struggle to make sure I was healing as I was sore, had engorged breasts and was sleep deprived. I didn't want to go back to the hospital or see a doctor. Surviving these days on my own with a new baby was one of the hardest things I have ever done. Thankfully my mom came to stay with me on day five.

A new mom should never be told that her child needs medical care, but cannot receive it. Before I left the NICU, I was notified that my girl needed to see an audio specialist, but the specialist had to stay home with her kids because the schools were shut down. Baby needed physiotherapy on her foot and shoulder but all the clinics were closed. The only medical professional I was able to see was a home nurse, and she was doing the job of all the medical personnel. At the time I was so scared because I couldn't provide enough care or receive the correct care for my baby.

A year later, my baby girl is healthy, happy, and loved. The year was full of many tears of anger, frustration, and the loss of all the first-time mom experiences I didn't get to have. But I was blessed to have had a drive-by baby shower, a campfire in the driveway for baby's first birthday, and so much love and support from friends and family. Many of my friends have not held the baby yet because the restrictions are still in place. But this alone time has strengthened my bond with my baby.

I am very proud to be a single mother by choice. My heart bursts every time I look at my girl. I'm still frequently asked; "how do you do it?" My answer is; "all you really need is love."

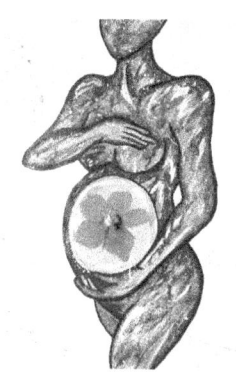

# REFLECTIONS ON PARENTING

# Arrival

*By Nadia Pestrak*

*Nadia recently moved to rural Ontario, where she lives with her two sons, dog, cat, and chickens.*

**Cigars**

I found an old cigar box colonized by my childhood. Inside were dozens of small paper dolls that I had drawn and coloured and carefully cut out, their bodies smudged and folded and worn from hours of play. Children, mothers with long skirts and curly hair, and fathers sporting moustaches. I pull at the pile of paper limbs and unloose a mama doll who, Pompeii-like, still holds in her carefully folded paper arms a baby.

**The Best of Intentions**

The day after a beautiful wedding in the Polish mountains, a group of us go for a hike. I walk alongside a new friend, our feet turning stones. I tell her about my plan, still testing the words out as well as my own conviction. I will have a child by myself. And if that doesn't work, I will adopt. If I can't adopt, I will foster. I will do anything short of kidnapping to be a mother. She, with two children of her own, asks kindly, earnestly, Why don't you just get a dog?

**Deer**

We are in the country. My mother is bent over her flowerbeds, pulling weeds out. I tell her, If I am 38 and I haven't met anyone I will have a baby on my own. She stands up straight, her face flushed from bending, opens her arms wide for an embrace, Bravo! As if I had accomplished something very fine. I may still meet someone, I remind her. If, I say, if, still in her embrace.

A few minutes later we look down towards the edge of the pond. A deer stands there, still, alert, ready. My mother looks at me with delight, as though it is my doing; my announcement has summoned this beauty.

**Arriving, despite.**

I was sure that my father would disapprove, and I didn't want to have to justify a path that at times had been painful to forge. I decided to say nothing.

Driving me to the airport at the end of a visit, my father tells me that he heard about my plan, supports me and understands that motherhood is an important part of who I am. He feels strongly and speaks warmly, and while he's talking, he gets distracted and takes a ramp to the wrong terminal. Damn it, he says, We have time though, don't worry. His words slow as he squints and considers the various lanes before us. And don't worry about meeting someone later on, he says, as we loop around and finally pull up in front of glass doors that open and close, travelers streaming into the building. This will bring out the best in you. The right person will see that. You'll end up where you want to be, even if it's not the way you expected to get there.

**Questions**

I read books about becoming a single mum by choice. In

one book there is a list of questions to help you determine your readiness. Have you grieved the loss of the family/partner you imagined you'd have? I am not sure. The boyfriend of many years, the one I most loved, my first love, who travelled with me on trains and buses for months, who knew me best of all, who remains tangled in songs and memories. Is there a way our path might have led to family? If I had found a way to release him, might I have met someone else? Have I grieved the loss of the partner I imagined I'd have? I am not sure.

But to the question, do you want to have a baby even on your worst of days? Yes, always, yes.

**The algorithm of online shopping:**

> Canadian-compliant sperm from a U.S. sperm bank
>
> Open donor (can be contacted when my child is 19)
>
> Rh negative (as I am)
>
> Any ethnicity
>
> A photo that, were it on an online dating site, would make me consider meeting in person (I have some faith in chemistry)
>
> An essay that I could feel good about the child having in their back pocket, "do not be afraid to seek me out, I will open my heart to you."

+ A good gut feeling

---

= **DONOR AGL5\*\*7**

**Unresolved**

Never has 'nature versus nurture' seemed so critical. I look at my donor's information. His SAT scores, his favorite books, the occupations of his parents and grandparents. What is the collection of genetic predispositions that supports someone living well in the world? Will my child want to contact the donor? What happens when Donor AGL5**7's phone rings again, for the 5th or 16th or 30th time? Will he be kind, even if he sold his sperm to get through school, even if he has a family of his own? Will he, in fact, open his heart when my child seeks him out?

**Trying**

After each insemination at the clinic (there are four), I have sex sometime during the 72 hours the sperm could survive. I am hoping the trysts will help my body grow a baby. The men don't know that I have migrated from that hard white bed and tunelessly humming doctor at the clinic, to their skin against mine, their sweat and the semblance of tenderness between us.

**Helium Balloons**

Two weeks after my fourth attempt there is spotting. It didn't work. At the end of the day I go for farewell drinks for a colleague. I throw up in the morning from too many shots, and the helium balloons I took from a pub are nodding heads against the ceiling. In the evening, out with an ex-boyfriend, the blood has not come. I do a pregnancy test in a movie theatre bathroom stall while my date waits with his buttered popcorn.

I return to the seat just as the theatre darkens. I sit with my secret and I feel my blood rise to the surface, warm my body, feel the most delectable excitement I've ever encountered, like so many fireflies rising in the darkness, like balloons.

**What I am Making**

I feel as though everything I experience when pregnant filters through in some way to my baby. I want to see beautiful paintings, look at the trees and sky. I want to hear only music I love. I want to be around people that make me laugh.

I follow my baby's progress with attention. My baby does not have a tail anymore. My baby can taste, my baby can hear. I read Rumi, Rilke, Song of Songs. I let the water from the shower drum lightly on my stomach, like the sound of rain on the roof. I swim, submerge, hear perhaps the sounds my baby hears. I will drop into beautiful things and rise back up with a baby.

## Expecting

The expectation for love and all that followed was always there. At five, I arranged marriages between my stuffed animals. At seven, I put dolls down to nap in dark rooms. When I was eight, my diary read of a boy at school: Today Ian leaned over to whisper something in my ear. I thought he would say, 'I love you,' but instead he whispered, 'Dana's a spaz.' Fourteen, I sat on my grandmother's roof at night. The sky was wide with stars and there were people going into the town across the harbor. I imagined them, moving through their adult nights, drunk, happy, desiring.

An unforeseen freedom arrives when I get pregnant. For the first time in my life I stop assuming that I am going to meet someone. Is that attractive man in the coffee line making an amiable comment to me? There is no need to impress, awkwardness is irrelevant; there are no possibilities to thwart.

## Let Me Run Again

The belly blooms. The body is a garden, fertile, thick and green and lush. All is promise, fat lilacs suffusing a summer garden with their gentle scent.

But it's a wayward garden. I learn that with the glow and bloom are aches and an inability to move fluidly. There is incontinence and flatulence and I struggle with socks. I am surprised at the body's many small betrayals.

I see a woman running; flushed, sweating, her thigh muscles taut, and I recall the exhilaration of movement. I remember the point at which the run shifts from granular to smooth and stamina arrives. I miss it with nostalgia entirely unfamiliar, as though it is an experience I will never again know, and I think, oh, yes, this is what is to come later. I meet the eyes of an elderly woman, walking very slowly on the street, as though in kinship.

**Animal Waiting**

In my final weeks, I am afraid to go out after dark. I know that this is unlike me, but there are strange inclinations these days. I long for old boyfriends and wake missing them like they have left their scent about me in the sheets. I miss the one I loved the most. His equanimity, his voice, the things we laughed at together, the alphabet of his facial expressions and the language only we knew. I must not be out in the snow, surrounded by blurred flashing red lights, the dark cold of winter night, alone.

**God Heals, Rafael**

When I think about luminous moments in my life, they are often small, unexpected – listening to a taxi driver talk about disappointment, Sibelius on the radio, the golden glow of a passing window revealing a room full of people doing Tai Chi, beautifully, impossibly coordinated. A blast of smoke on a ferry in Bangkok, my body against strangers, sweat dripping down my back, the boat thrumming on the beige river. A deer standing alert at the edge of a pond.

Obvious though it is, my joy has never been so expansive and undiluted: your bright red starfish limbs, held in the air, here, at last, coming to rest on my belly. I will return to this, remembering, here, here, when I am that old woman on the sidewalk passing someone pregnant, remembering, when the longing of youth, that city I sought on the horizon, is a distant constellation of lights. I will remember again the surprise of your blood-and-mucus-covered beauty, the end of the pain, arrival, at last.

# Crazy or Brave? Single and Trying for a Second Child

*By Athena Reich*

*Athena is an actress, singer/songwriter, writer, and world renowned Lady Gaga Impersonator. Her son plays "Hudson" in Netflix's "Sex/Life" and her journey to conceive through IVF is featured in the Emmy nominated documentary "Vegas Baby." www.AthenaReich.com.*

I wrote this piece originally for pregnantish.com when I was on the brink of trying for my second child as a solo mom. Catch up with me now, at the end of the piece, to see how it all turned out!

---

Am I overly ambitious or heart-driven? I can't settle on whether trying to have a second child, as a single mother by choice, is logical – or naïve.

But I am pursuing this path anyway, because although I have a wonderful, beautiful little boy, I really want – have always wanted – two children. I have also always wanted a partner, but when my girlfriend and I broke up when I was 36, I knew it was time to pursue parenthood on my own. A heart can wait, but egg quality – not so much.

After numerous IUI and IVF attempts, I gave birth to my

son using egg and sperm donation. He is now three years old, and I have just begun estrogen in preparation for the transfer of new embryos (created with the same sperm, but new eggs; as my son's egg donor retired).

I have spent the past year obsessing whether I should continue to build my family. Ever since I was a little girl I wanted two children or more – five, even! I remember daydreaming about my mom having a third or that I had a secret twin on the other side of the world. Maybe it's because all of my relatives live in another country, or because my parents split when I was five, but I always longed for my own little tribe. However, this was all under the assumption that I would be married.

Of course, it's hard to ignore the sensible idioms: "Don't bite off more than you can chew," "Quit while you're ahead," and "Be grateful for what you have." Logically I agree it would be simpler to not have a second.

What has my experience of motherhood been like so far, especially after waiting and fighting so hard to become a mom? Similar to practically every other mother: it's harder than I imagined, unrelentingly exhausting, irritating, frustrating, and yet, more often than not, packed with gorgeous sweetness, multiple times per day. Motherhood fills my life with undeniable meaning and depth.

Over the past year, I tried over and over to imagine stopping at one child but no matter how I looked at it, it felt like defeat. Maybe when it comes to big life decisions, the analytical brain shouldn't win. Maybe when it comes to love, children, and big life goals, you've got to follow your heart. "Where there's a will there's a way" and "Follow your passion" are the phrases that come to mind now. (I guess there's a saying for every side of an argument.)

So here I am, taking birth control again, in preparation for an embryo transfer. Yet, I still feel mixed about it. Or maybe vulnerable is a better word.

Yesterday I sobbed on my mother's couch, unloading about ten million concerns – from how to juggle everything with my demanding career, to my lack of confidence as a mother, to whether this new transfer will work, to plain terror about taking on a second child at a time when my first just started letting me empty the dishwasher without screaming to be picked up.

My mom listened empathetically, and when I mentioned I just got my period and started birth control, she said, "A-ha…" We laughed because every month I do seem to come to her crying about ten million things, right on schedule, especially when there's extra estrogen involved.

And what about love and marriage? I do feel I am missing out. Of course, it would be amazing to feel like someone "gets" me, adores me, and could reassure me that I'm sexy, a great mom, and that we can take on anything as a couple because our love is strong and our finances double!

But I also know that relationships can sometimes be disappointing and painful, especially when children are involved. Maybe I'm not worse off as a single mom… I do, however, get lonely sometimes.

Lately I've been foraging into a world I thought I left long ago, the world of casual sex – with men! Even though I'm a lesbian, there's something about baby-making (and perhaps extra estrogen) that makes me want to have sex with men. Casual sex with men is easy for me, because I don't want a relationship afterwards.

Casual sex with women, on the other hand, is more fraught because I fall in love so easily. And, as someone who is creating a baby, it's ironically a terrible time to start a relationship. I can't imagine expending that energy, while parenting a preschooler, trying to create a human, and then (hopefully) breastfeeding 'round the clock.

Also, from a legal standpoint, starting a long term relationship while pursuing parenthood could get challenging. Procreating for lesbians involves using reproductive technologies, so if I was with a woman for a couple of years and we had a nasty break-up she could unfortunately argue that because she was there during the baby-making process, she is a parent. I realize that with every new love comes risk, but if I wait for love until after my family is created, it's clear that I am the intended parent. Of course, had I found love years ago and created children with a wife, I would have been willing to take that risk. But developing a relationship right in the middle of family-building doesn't seem wise to me.

However… if an incredibly empathetic and patient woman suddenly emerges who is absolutely perfect, I would be open to it. But since I'm not on the lookout, casual sex is the most practical (and yes, fun) option at the moment. It satisfies my desire for physical contact, though I know there is still risk, both physically (I practice safe sex but you still wonder) and emotionally (it can take up some time and energy to process).

Yes, I've got mixed feelings about a lot of things. But after talking to my circle of married moms, it seems I am not alone in experiencing the excitement, the fear, the panic, and the daydreaming (of what my little baby girl or boy might be like), when considering a second.

Single or not, it seems common to be scared of mothering another. As a single woman though, people question me a lot more, and, when you are shelling out tens of thousands of dollars (or more!) for artificial reproductive technology, and bringing yourself to the clinic for regular ultrasounds and blood draws, you have more time to overthink things.

Could the embryo fairy please just fly into my womb, and then I can tell everyone I had no choice... it was Immaculate Conception!?

Could the most perfect woman on the planet please just appear? She will be full of understanding and patience, and we can get to know each at a safe snail's pace while I conceive, so that nothing is risked or rushed?

Could this next transfer please work so I can save myself the ups and downs I know all too well as someone who suffered through many IUI's and IVF's to create my first?

Yes, I am a dreamer, but a goal-oriented one. Although the waves of anxiety roll in and out, I am determined to create my own special family. I've always wanted my own little pack and it is my main priority now. I have got to believe that when the right woman comes along, she will share my dream of family, and it will all work out.

---

**Three Years Later**

My preschooler is now starting Grade One and my much-longed-for second born is a strong, gorgeous, talkative, brilliant and willful two-year-old girl. I am writing this update from Tamarindo in Costa Rica, where I have run away for a few months (after getting my two Pfizer jabs) to work remotely, take in sunsets on the beach, enroll my children in fantastic jungle camps and get a break from the past two years of COVID-19 Hell.

As a solo mom, I have much to say about how the Canadian government disregarded single parents during the pandemic, and did not do a targeted enough approach to Covid-19 prevention; thus harming families, working moms and the mental health of children. However, this piece is not about the world. It's about a (perhaps) brave, yet terrifying, choice to have two children on my own and I'm sure you are all wondering how it played out.

Is it hard? You bet. Extremely. I'm tired. Last night my toddler screamed for hours because I am trying to night-wean her. Both kids want me all the time, and I am definitely out-numbered. In the first year it was almost unbearably difficult. I discovered my eldest has ADHD and his moods, jealousy and tantrums were practically too much to handle with a newborn. However, the more my daughter grew, the more my son started having fun with her. Now they entertain each other (thank God – finally) and the love they have for each other is utterly irreplaceable. I have no regrets now as I love them both so much, and we do feel like the little tribe I always longed for.

The only advice I would give, if you are considering making this choice, is to earn as much money as you possibly can because you need to spend a large chunk of it on childcare. (If you are in the lucky position of having family or friends with time on their hands – in my opinion you have won the lottery so please disregard this advice!) In my situation, however, and with so many others, we need the extra help. Right now, in addition to daycare and camp, I have someone helping me in the early evenings with dinner, clean-up and splitting attention between my two very young kids. I am a better parent and my anxiety level lowers a few notches just knowing I'm not going to be alone with two fussy youngsters at the end of my work day.

The nuclear family is a construct. I am reminded of this each time my married friends have profound complaints about their spouses, or announce another divorce. And the breakdown of the extended family, consisting of grandparents, aunts and cousins nearby, has created an urgent childcare deficit, one that most often falls on the shoulders of women. It always took a village and choosing to be a solo mom is a wonderful choice — just know that you will most likely need to find, or pay, for a lot of help. And even if you can't, or choose to DO IT ALL on your own, you will survive, and it is all, most certainly, worth it.

And in regards to dating? I have not had time and the damn pandemic has made new romance nearly impossible. I hope that soon, as things continue to open up, I can go on regular dates and start working on my next life goal; a happy marriage that fits beautifully (enough) into my dream of being a mom.

If you want kids, and you are single, I say do it.

Maybe I will create my own idiom. Something along the lines of; "Follow your heart and the path will follow." Logic, be damned. As the Dalai Lama XIV says, "Choose to be optimistic. It feels better."

# Finding My Power in Motherhood

*by Myriam Steinberg*

*Myriam is currently a writer and grateful mother to twins. Her first book,* Catalogue Baby: A Memoir of (In)fertility, *chronicles her years spent trying to conceive a child as a single woman in her forties. www.cataloguebabynovel.com.*

After years of infertility and fetal loss of various kinds, I became a Single Mother by Choice to a set of beautiful twins. The journey to becoming a parent was an excruciatingly physical and emotional experience. As the years of trying to conceive dragged on, I was living with the devastation of seeing my body betray me and my dreams of family life being shattered as I struggled to get pregnant, and when I did, seeing one baby after another leave my body well before its time. I also, as with many people who have decided to become Single Mothers by Choice in their later years, had other pieces of baggage added on to my already tall pile of insecurities and grief.

For me, that extra luggage consisted of two giant suitcases: The first was "How did I let my career of running a festival take over my life in such an all-consuming way?" The second was "What's wrong about me as a person that I am chronically single?"

When I finally decided to shut the festival down, it took over a year for me to recover, somewhat, from the intense burnout and loss of identity I'd experienced in the final years of running it. The drive to have children was so strong however, that before that year was out, and despite still healing from the burnout, I decided to begin trying to get pregnant. I figured having a successful birth would be part of my recovery process. On top of that, the consequences of sacrificing everything for my career served to fuel my urgency at trying to conceive a child.

The second issue I came to terms with by telling myself: "People with children meet their significant others just as well as people without kids." Even more importantly, if I have a kid, there won't be any more procreation pressure placed on whatever intimate relationship I might pursue. I would be in the relationship for the right reasons: that we were truly compatible, that the person I was with was kind, intelligent, interesting, funny, and yes, good in bed. It wouldn't just be because "they like me, we basically get along, and I want a child." The moment I realized this, the "need" to find a partner completely dissolved and I went from feeling like I was a Single Mother by Unfortunate Circumstance to being a Single Mother by Choice. This completely took off the pressure for me to try and meet someone and allowed me to focus on my goal of having children.

In retrospect, undergoing the quest for motherhood as a single person was indeed the best thing that could have happened. With my difficult journey, I can't imagine having to mitigate another person's grief as I was trying to survive my own. I can't imagine having to negotiate what the stop-point would be in the quest for children. What if theirs was significantly different than mine? Would that have meant the end of that relationship and I'd be right where I was anyways – a single woman trying to have a viable pregnancy that would result in the birth of a living, healthy child?

Would that have meant stopping well before I was ready to? I already had to endure comments of "Perhaps it wasn't meant to be and you should move on?" from well-meaning friends and some family. I couldn't have borne it if it also came from my partner.

In going it alone, I have gained a confidence and strength in the power of my own voice and will that I never had before. Any relationship I am in must be good for not just me, but the children as well. That means that the kids always come first, and they serve as a kind of filter for the good and the bad. They force me to voice my opinions, desires, and choices loudly, clearly, and unambiguously.

People talk about the "loss of self" that often goes along with having children. For me, however, having children has enriched my identity. I feel like I have found myself. My role as a mother does not mean that I am subsuming myself to the needs of my children. Fulfilling their needs, and keeping them alive, healthy, and happy, only demonstrates the strength and resilience I am capable of. Living life as a mom and as a creative, useful member of society, takes some juggling but they are both equally important to me. So I strive for both, and don't sweat the small stuff in order to achieve that.

I went from mourning the loss of a partner to celebrating the courage and fortitude I had in pursuing my dreams of creating a family. I am no longer putting myself second. If someone wants to join me on my path, and they are the right person, they are welcome – on my terms.

It is an extraordinary place to be.

# Resource List

If you are interested in choice parenting and want to learn more, here are a few places you can start.

**Books**

- *Catalogue Baby: A Memoir of (In)Fertility* by Myriam Steinberg. A tragicomic graphic memoir about a single woman's attempts to conceive in her 40s. And, she just so happens to be featured in this anthology.

- *Do I Want to Be a Mom?* by Diana Dell and Suzan Erem. Co-written by one woman who chose to have children, and another woman who chose not to. Thought-provoking and helpful, if you're on the fence.

- *Choosing Single Motherhood: A Thinking Woman's Guide* by Mikki Morrissette. Intended as a comprehensive guide.

- *Single Mothers by Choice: A Guidebook for Single Women Who Are Considering or Have Chosen Motherhood* by Jane Mattes. Written in 1994 – a classic read, though dated in parts.

- *Knock Yourself Up* by Louise Sloan. A US-based single mother by choice who tells it all on her journey. Not for everyone, but worth checking out.

- *Going Solo* by Genevieve Roberts

- *Single by Chance, Mothers by Choice: How women are choosing parenthood without marriage and creating the new American family* by Rosanna Hertz (2006)

- *An excellent choice. Panic and joy on my solo path to motherhood* by Emma Brockes (2018)

**Podcasts**

- Not by Accident – story of an Australian woman who becomes a single parent by choice while living in Europe

- Choice Chat podcast – a whole range of topics from fertility, to navigating donors, to single parenting.

- The Single Greatest Choice

- Mocha SMC

- Sperm Cast

- The Stork and I

- Motherhood Reimagined

**Websites to start with**

- www.singlemothersbychoice.org

- www.choicemoms.org

- www.choosingsingleparenthood.com

**Facebook Groups**

- Single Mothers by Choice Canada

- Queer Single Parents by Choice

- Single Moms by Choice Travel

- Choice Moms in Vancouver, Choice Parents Toronto, and other city-based and regional groups.

www.ingramcontent.com/pod-product-compliance
Lightning Source LLC
Chambersburg PA
CBHW071421070526
44578CB00003B/644